Holding the Ball

How I Survived Pelvic Organ Prolapse - Without Surgery!

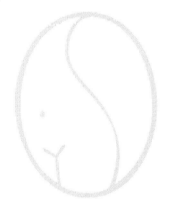

Julia F. Kaye

Waye Forward (Publishing) Ltd
Llanishen
Cardiff
CF14 5FA

ISBN-13: 9780993087707
ISBN-10: 0993087701

Cover Design: Claire Cater

MEDICAL DISCLAIMER

The information provided in this publication is not intended to be a substitute for professional medical advice, diagnosis or treatment. You are advised to seek medical support if you are affected by the issues raised in this book. Do not disregard professional medical advice, or delay in seeking it, because of something you have read here. Do not rely on information in this publication in place of seeking professional medical advice.

This publication is for information only. After reading the book, you are encouraged to review the information carefully with your professional healthcare provider.

PERSONAL DISCLAIMER

I am not a doctor or healthcare professional. The information I provide is based on my personal experience, thorough secondary research, and conversations with other women who have experienced pelvic organ prolapse or related conditions. Any recommendations I make about self-help or lifestyle changes should be discussed between you and your professional healthcare provider.

CONTENTS

ABOUT THE AUTHOR

Julia Kaye has an Honours Degree in English and a PGCE from Leicester University. Her background is in teaching and charity administration, and she is currently a co-director of two small companies.

She has appeared on BBC TV's 'The One Show' as a case study for managing depression through exercise (May 2008), and been interviewed by HTV News and BBC Radio 4 for documentary features on the lived experience of depression.

Julia has a track record in emerging from personal misfortune to feel inspired by it and driven towards helping others to manage (or even avoid) a similar situation themselves. She developed and shared her own "tool kit" of self-help strategies to use alongside medical support to combat depression; and having recently experienced and managed pelvic organ prolapse, she set up a website for women giving information and advice about preventing and managing POP at www.womensbits.org

Her recent experience of pelvic organ prolapse has also been the trigger for writing this book. in which she shares with the reader her progress through recovery, and the self-help techniques she learned and made part of her life in order to manage her condition.

Julia lives in Cardiff with her husband Nick, and has two grown-up children.

ACKNOWLEDGMENTS

Thanks go to Carole Broad for pelvic floor muscle training; to Pam Henley who signposted me towards gynaecological physiotherapy; to Mary Madhavi of www.marysyoga.com and www.yogamobility.org for yoga, cranio-sacral therapy, and counselling which helped me to manage and overcome my pelvic organ prolapse; to Tim Watkins for design, illustrations, typesetting, and encouragement; to Simon Turney for proof-reading; and to Nick Kaye for photography, but most of all for his loving support.

FOREWORD

This book has been written as a direct result of personal experience. I was diagnosed with prolapse of the uterus and bladder in December 2010 and have managed to overcome this without surgery - even though two GP's and a gynaecology consultant were all pointing me in this direction, and offering a vaginal ring pessary as the only other option. I have been spared much misery and trauma by sheer luck, through having had the right people around me; my yoga teacher (a trained counsellor) who helped me work through the emotional issues, and a friend who told me about gynaecological physiotherapy and suggested that I insist on being referred for this treatment.

Currently in the UK most women with prolapse are prescribed a pessary, or directed towards surgery - an expensive option which only has a sixty to eighty per cent success rate. Either of these treatments can trigger further problems.

If physiotherapy and emotional support were made routinely available to all women diagnosed with pelvic organ prolapse in the UK, the number of women who would benefit is huge: the NHS reports that one third of women in the UK are affected by some form of pelvic organ prolapse. Many of these will be over fifty but younger women are also affected, as is shown by the numbers of women in their forties, thirties, and even twenties using women's online forums to express their anxieties about prolapse-related symptoms.

I should like to see women diagnosed with pelvic organ prolapse offered gynaecological physiotherapy in the first instance, with surgery being the last resort. The emotional impact of prolapse also needs to be recognised, with access to free counselling forming part of the treatment programme.

Meanwhile, whatever treatment is offered involves a waiting list to access it, and then takes time to become effective. During the time I spent waiting, I discovered ways and means of managing my condition both physically and emotionally, and reducing its impact on my daily life and wellbeing. I share these self-help techniques with you throughout this book, and you will also find them highlighted at the end of each relevant chapter, along with key information about POP for quick and easy reference.

Julia Kaye - 2014

Chapter 1

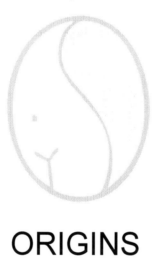

ORIGINS

ORIGINS

It was a week before Christmas 2011, and there had been exceptionally heavy snowfall throughout the country. The nights were unusually cold, and any slight thaw during daylight hours turned to ice after dark. Drivers were abandoning their cars on the side of the roads or leaving them where they had parked them earlier in the day. People were cancelling social events, and many were working from home.

I had spent the weekend in a very sedentary fashion, sitting at my computer or at the dining-room table wrapping presents and writing cards. I was feeling a bit sore in the area my daughter used to refer to (when she was a little girl) as her "front bottom", but I put this discomfort down to sitting in the same position for too long, in jeans which had (somehow!) got a bit tight since the summer months.

The soreness persisted beyond the weekend, despite swapping the tight jeans for comfortable leggings. Something was not right. I investigated, gently feeling inside with my fingers. There was a large, soft swelling on the upper wall of my vagina. What could this be? I logged on to the NHS Direct website and keyed in my symptoms, hoping to find something reassuring......

The advice there was that I should see a doctor within thirty-six hours.

I phoned the surgery. The receptionist told me there were no appointments available; but when I described the problem and the NHS Direct advice she was more accommodating and was able to give me an appointment with a female doctor that afternoon.

There had been no improvement in the weather. On the contrary, there had been another heavy fall of snow which now lay in a thick layer over all the pathways that many people had worked so stalwartly over the weekend to clear. Beneath the new snow, the old snow was packed down hard and unyielding, a hazardous under-layer of ice. My snow-covered car had been parked in the drive for four days, and was not going anywhere.

Fortunately, the surgery was not far away. But the short walk seemed a challenging distance. Walking had always been one of my pleasures, but not this time. I was frightened of falling. I did not yet have a diagnosis, but I knew instinctively that slipping over on the ice and landing heavily would probably make matters worse. When had I last felt so physically vulnerable? When I was pregnant, perhaps? At fifty-nine I felt like an old lady, gingerly feeling my way forward step by step.

I made it to the surgery and saw the GP. She diagnosed a prolapsed uterus. My womb had slipped downwards, out of place. This happens, as she explained, in forty to fifty per cent of women over the age of forty, particularly those who have given birth vaginally. I was already thinking, "That's an awful lot of women. And it happens particularly to women who give birth naturally? That seems a cruel twist of fate to me! And it happens to so many of us... if that's so, why has nobody mentioned this to me before?"

The GP was still speaking to me. I tuned back in, trying to focus. She was saying that I would probably need surgery to support the uterus. The ultimate would be a hysterectomy, though she did not recommend this as the vagina that remains behind can then prolapse too. She promised to refer me to a specialist, though she warned that it would be a few months before I got an appointment (and, of course, many more months after that before I would be treated).

I felt sick, shocked and shaky as if I had been slapped, though the doctor's manner was nothing but kind. It could not be me that she was talking to! I had always been pretty well physically, quite fit even. Did I hear the word *surgery*? Did I hear the word *specialist*? It could not be me.

"Listen! Focus!" I told myself. "I am being given some advice to help me manage this".

I was to tighten my pelvic floor muscles twenty-five times a day. I was to avoid standing for long spells. Again I could feel old age creeping over me, as if I was suddenly turning into the old lady that I would normally have given up my seat for on the bus. I was not to strain on the toilet, so no pushing to poo. I was not to lift anything heavy. (How heavy was heavy?) Gentle exercise, like walking, cycling, swimming or yoga, would be good for me as it would help to tone the muscles.

So I could go for a walk, but not lift a rucksack. I could go for a bike ride, as long as I did not haul my bike around at all. I could still do yoga, but not on my own as I was not sure whether I could do all my usual postures safely. I could go for a swim..... I hated swimming.

But I just had to accept all this, because it was indeed *me* that she was talking to.

KEY INFORMATION

Pelvic Organ Prolapse can happen suddenly without any obvious warning

It is common in women over forty

It is treatable

If you suspect that something has happened to your womb, bladder, bowel and/or vagina it is important to see your doctor without delay

SELF-HELP TIPS

straining the bowel or standing up for a long time are not advised when you have POP

Exercising the pelvic floor is essential to managing POP

Gentle exercise like walking, cycling, swimming or yoga is recommended

For more information about POP and how to manage it – read on!

Chapter 2

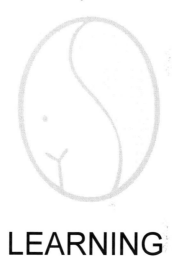

LEARNING

LEARNING

It could have been worse, of course. The diagnosis was not life-threatening. But my condition could be life-*changing*, and not in a good way. I needed to feel that I had some control over the situation. To have even a semblance of control, I needed to know more about the condition. So I searched the Internet for more information.

Diagram of the female pelvic floor

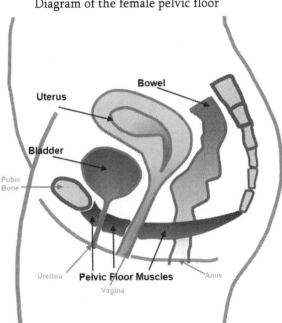

I learned that there are various forms of prolapse of the pelvic organs (uterus, bladder, and bowel), known collectively as pelvic organ prolapse. "To prolapse" means to fall down, so medically the word prolapse describes a sinking downwards of the womb (uterus), the bladder, and/or the lower bowel (rectum).

The most common form is uterine prolapse, where the womb slips down into the vagina, even becoming visible at or below the vaginal opening. Prolapse of the bladder, where the bladder slips downwards and presses into the front of the vaginal wall, is called cystocele (pronounced *sis-te-seel*). Prolapse of the rectum, where the lower bowel presses into the back of the vaginal wall, is called rectocele (pronounced *rec-te-seel*). Pelvic organ prolapse causes pressure on the vagina such that the vagina prolapses as well to some degree, the vaginal wall sinking inwards and downwards towards the vaginal opening. In more severe cases, the prolapsed organ herniates (i.e. pushes) through the vaginal wall.

Pelvic organ prolapse is caused by activities or events that put pressure on the pelvic floor muscle at the base of the pelvis (hip bone) which supports these organs. This is a large group of muscle fibres which extends from the pubis at the front of the body to the base of the spine at the back. It is the muscle you contract when you want to stop yourself from passing wee, poo, or wind. Even more important, it is literally the 'floor' of your body, upon which all the organs within the pelvis rest. Your womb, bladder, and intestine are all held in place by your pelvic floor, and by very little else apart from connective tissue. So you can see how important it is to look after your pelvic floor and keep it strong. It has a great deal of work to do.

I found that the most prevalent causes of pelvic organ prolapse are the following, which all put pressure on the pelvic floor:

o   being pregnant in the later stages, especially with a large baby (or more than one)

o   having a baby via the birth canal (vagina), especially more than once, with little recovery time between pregnancies

o   high impact exercise, such as running, aerobics, or jumping (e.g. skipping, trampoline, circuit training)

o   abdominal exercises, such as sit-ups or crunches

o   lifting a heavy weight – for instance, a young child

o   being overweight for a long time

o   constipation, i.e. straining to poo

o   having a persistent cough.

As these factors are relevant to women of all ages, pelvic organ prolapse can affect women of all ages too. But time is also a factor, making older women even more at risk due to muscular weakness and hormonal changes.

According to the BBC Health website, as many as half of all women who have given birth twice or more will have some form of pelvic organ prolapse at a later stage. About one in every eight women over forty is likely to have some degree of uterine prolapse. The NHS reports that one third of adult women in the UK are affected by some form of pelvic organ prolapse.

Reading the information I found about the signs and symptoms of POP was an eye-opener, as I recognised some of them. With hindsight I realised that I should have known that all was not well.

Early warning signs of pelvic organ prolapse include:

o   pain in the lower back, or a sense of stiffness or weakness there
o   occasional leakage from the bladder (stress incontinence) or the bowel
o   vaginal bleeding or discharge
o   pain or discomfort during sex.

Symptoms of POP include:

o   a feeling in the vagina as if a ball is coming down it, or as if there is something heavy there
o   swelling in the vaginal wall

o   urge incontinence (a sudden need to rush to the loo to pass urine, so sudden that you might not make it in time)

o   a feeling that the bladder is not emptying properly

o   difficulty passing stools

o   a dragging sensation in the pelvic area, similar to the feeling of being heavily pregnant, or having a very heavy period

o   in severe cases, the prolapsed organ (e.g. the cervix or uterus) or the bulging vaginal wall may be visible beyond the vaginal opening.

Needless to say, if reading this information (or any other part of this book) raises for you any concerns about your own health, it is important that you see your doctor without delay.

Reading all this made me feel a bit better informed. All the same, the more facts I picked up, the more I realised that the inside of my own body was a mystery to me. I had thought that I knew about human biology. Now it was as if I had known nothing at all. I looked at diagrams of the female pelvic structure and could make no sense of them, because what I saw bore no relation to how I was feeling inside. I could not get a handle on where my uterus now was, or where it was supposed to be in relation to everything else. Was it pressing on my bladder? Was that the bulge that I could feel in the vaginal wall? And if my uterus had slipped downwards, what normally held it in place? And what did the pelvic floor muscle (which appeared as a thin line in the sideways-view diagrams I was studying) have to do with it all?

I felt very ignorant, and vulnerable. And I was feeling my age, which I rarely had up to that point; all of my fifty-nine years. It would have been comforting to turn to an older female relative and talk this through with someone who could reassure and advise; the Wise Woman of times gone by. But all these were gone; I was the matriarch now, feeling old but not wise.

I thought about those women in my family who had passed on. I remembered how my grandmother always used to rest with her feet up for an hour or so every afternoon. Did my grandmother have a prolapse? She had apparently rested like this since her late twenties:

"The doctor says I must," she used to say. "Never stand when you can sit, never sit when you can lie."

I used to think that that sounded lazy – but then, my grandmother was not a lazy person. On the contrary, she was busy and socially active well into her nineties. She had an odd way of walking too, and I wondered now whether there was more to that than just stiffness in her joints. But if she had a prolapse, she would never have spoken of it: that would have been most improper in her opinion. And no physical problems ever stopped her from being a strong, proactive, and elegant lady, even during her final years.

If only we could have talked of these things! She could have taught me so much, wisdom gathered over a life-time of experience! But as I thought about her I realised that in remembering her daily routines I was, in a sense, receiving her advice. Whether her early afternoon rest was related to prolapse or not, in future it would be a good idea to make it a part of my own lifestyle. I soon found that if I was on my feet for too long, my symptoms became much worse; the dragging sensation like the start of a period, and the swelling feeling as if something was trying to push its way out between my legs.

Sitting down reduced these symptoms, and lying down eased them significantly. But this presented me with a challenge. Being busy is my default position. I bustle about from one task to another, even having several on-going at the same time. No sooner have I sat down (say, to open the mail) than I am up again to fetch something I need, or write a post-it note, or look up a point of interest, or put the kettle on..... this bustling activity has irritated people close to me in the past, but I could never understand why. Now the issue became clear. I had been rushing about being busy to avoid sitting still. Sitting still is hard work. But now I was going to have to, if I was to manage this condition and not make it worse.

I worked at it. My first attempt at sitting down with my feet up on a stool was memorably difficult, fighting myself all the way. The urge to be up and about and faffing around on my feet was overwhelming. I sat for an hour battling my whizzing thoughts and rising agitation. But I remained with my feet up. Eventually I became calm enough and focused enough to sit and write down how I was feeling. Then I lay down on the settee to read.

If going through prolapse had a purpose, perhaps this was it for now – it was forcing me to take a good look at myself, and to slow down. I began to see that that busy, energetic person was only a part of who I am. I gave her permission to take a break and treat herself more gently. Sometimes she listened and responded: sometimes she rebelled. Sometimes she could be tricked into submission – sitting with her feet up by the window watching the birds bustling in the garden could satisfy the need to be busy, for a little while.

KEY INFORMATION

Prolapse can involve the womb, the bladder, and/or the bowel. It is caused by circumstances which put pressure on the pelvic floor, such as:

being pregnant in the later stages, especially with a large baby (or more than one)

having a baby via the birth canal (vagina), especially more than once, with little recovery time between pregnancies

high impact exercise, such as running, aerobics, or jumping (e.g. skipping, trampoline, circuit training)

abdominal exercises, such as sit-ups or crunches

lifting a heavy weight – for instance, a young child

being overweight for a long time

constipation, i.e. straining to poo

having a persistent cough.

Early warning signs of pelvic organ prolapse include:

pain in the lower back, or a sense of stiffness or weakness there occasional leakage from the bladder (stress incontinence) or the bowel

vaginal bleeding or discharge

pain or discomfort during sex

Symptoms of POP include:

a feeling in the vagina as if a ball is coming down it, or as if there is something heavy there

swelling in the vaginal wall

urge incontinence (a sudden need to rush to the loo to pass urine, so sudden that you might not make it in time)

a feeling that the bladder is not emptying properly

difficulty passing stools

a dragging sensation in the pelvic area, similar to the feeling of being heavily pregnant, or having a very heavy period

in severe cases, the prolapsed organ (e.g. the cervix or uterus) or the bulging vaginal wall may be visible beyond the vaginal opening.

Chapter 3

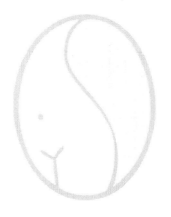

COPING,
YOGA-STYLE

Coping, Yoga-style

So it was going quite well, all things considered. I was finding out more about my condition, and learning to take things easy. I was able to manage the situation without having to talk about it outside my family. But that was Christmas, a time conducive to resting, reading and relaxation once all the festivities were over. Now it was January, and time to re-engage with the world outside. I felt like going into hiding instead.

I tried to push the prolapse issue to the back of my mind and get on with business as usual. But my back ached all the time, not only from the condition itself but also from the tension of trying to hold everything in (both physically and emotionally) and cringe away from it at the same time. Either I was going to have to confront my condition, or I was going to have to allow it to dominate me.

My first engagement of the New Year was at YogaMobility, a charity which runs yoga classes for people with physical and/or emotional challenges. For the previous few months I had been attending the classes as a helper. This time I was going as a participant...

Mary Madhavi, who founded YogaMobility in the 1970s, had been my yoga teacher, cranio-sacral therapist, mentor and friend for many years. She picked up that something was wrong as soon as she saw me, as I knew she would. What I did not know was that she had experienced pelvic organ prolapse herself. The advice she gave me that day, based on her knowledge, expertise and personal experience, was invaluable and well worth coming out of hiding for.

She suggested taking arnica tablets for a few days to reduce the inflammation she detected in my pelvic area; fish oil or flaxseed oil would also help, she said, and glucosamine and chondroitin to strengthen the connective tissue. I checked this out with the GP on my next visit to the surgery, and she agreed that these supplements could be beneficial, and would not do any me harm.

Mary also demonstrated some positions which could ease the symptoms, such as lying back on my elbows and, with my knees up, tilting my pelvis upwards.

She recommended the Shoulder Stand (*Salamba Sarvangasana*) as being particularly beneficial, because in this upside-down yoga posture the pelvic organs ease gently back into their natural positions: it reminds the body where they need to be. This posture also improves blood-flow into the abdominal area, which can promote healing. I began to hope that the stretched ligaments could actually be strengthened and mended.

"This position is so good for your condition," said Mary, "that you need to be putting your feet up for at least forty-five minutes every day."

"I'm trying to do that," I said.

"I don't just mean up," said Mary. "I mean *up*. Right up *in the air*."

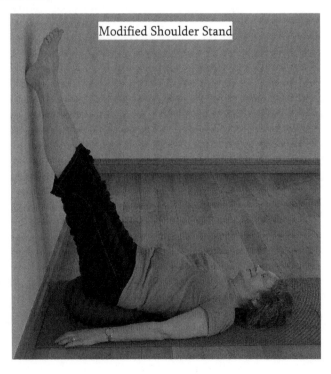

Modified Shoulder Stand

So I began to include a modified Shoulder Stand into my daily routine. The full Shoulder Stand was too uncomfortable for me, as I had been suffering from acid reflux (heartburn) for several months and this made my stomach too sensitive. But lying on my back with my bottom on a cushion (to tilt my pelvis upwards) and my feet in the air (or up against a wall) appeared to have a similar effect on my pelvic organs and noticeably took pressure off my pelvic floor.

Having struggled with the concept of putting my feet up in the conventional way, I actually found putting my feet right up in the air was much easier for me. Perhaps this was because I had to concentrate more, or perhaps because it was more difficult to leap up out of the position to get busy with something else. I focused on the things I could do in this position to pass the time. There were not many, but they were good enough. I could read a book, listen to music, look at the sky, or speak on the phone.....thank goodness Father Christmas had brought me a Kindle!

Besides the YogaMobility sessions, I went back to Mary's regular Yoga classes when they resumed in the New Year. I knew that with Mary as my teacher I was in safe hands. Besides the Shoulder Stand (or a modified version) she encouraged me to do the Pose of Eight Curves as well (part of the Sun Salutation sequence -

Surya Namaskar), as long as I felt comfortable, as she felt that this posture would be beneficial for me. I could do the Boat posture (*Navasana*) too if I felt strong enough, as this helps to strengthen core muscles including the pelvic floor. She advised against doing many vigorous breathing exercises for a while (*Kapalabhati* or *Bhastrika*), but suggested doing frequently a breathing exercise (*Mula Bandha*) that involves drawing up the pelvic floor and holding it there while holding a deep breath in (or out).

I was pleased to find that before long I could join in most of the class, as long as I was prepared to listen carefully to my body and respond to it. The basic rule was "If it feels uncomfortable, don't do it." This was a new experience for me, as I have always been a determined person, keen to push myself as far as possible to test my limits. But that kind of attitude would not help this time. There were occasions when I had to listen to Mary and do what she told me rather than what I wanted to do, but I had to accept that at those times she could "read" my body better than I could, and better understand its needs.

So I learned to do the Cat Stretch posture (*Biliasana*) without tilting my pelvis too far down, and to bend my legs in forward-bend postures (either sitting or standing). Sitting postures were made easier by sitting on a wedge-shaped cushion or by using a specially designed yoga back-rest called a backjack.

I had to accept that I could not bend sideways or backwards very far. I could still do side-bend postures like the Triangle (*Trikonasana*) and back-bend postures like the Cobra (*Bhujangasana*) with care and under Mary's watchful eye, bending only as far as was comfortable and no further. Some days I could hardly move at all: other days it was easier. My ability or lack of it was not always predictable.

Mary advised me not to attempt full back-bend postures like the Wheel (*Chakrasana*) or the Bow (*Dhanurasana*). While the rest of the class were doing these I would go into Cat Stretch position, then raise and stretch out my right arm forwards and my left leg back, before switching to do the same with my left arm and right leg, alternating these movements to keep up the work on my core muscles.

All this kept me moving. But I was learning to accept that when my body started to feel tired I needed to respect it and let it take a break, rather than push myself to do more.

I was disappointed at first to find that relaxing flat on the floor in the Corpse posture (*Savasana*) at the end of the asana (movement) sessions was uncomfortable, but placing a large cushion under my knees solved that problem. Placing a wedge under my bottom to tilt my pelvis up a bit was even more effective.

Thus I was able to continue with my regular yoga practice in this modified form, much to my relief. As far as I am concerned, it is the most important form of exercise that I do. I have practised yoga for the past ten years, and have found it hugely beneficial for both my physical and emotional wellbeing.

However, I cannot overstate the importance of finding and working with an experienced and well-qualified teacher if you want to try yoga yourself, especially if you have a health condition such as POP. If you are just thinking of taking up yoga as a preventative measure to maintain a strong pelvic floor then I suggest that you check out yoga classes in your area, and read up on yoga postures to get an idea of what is involved. The physical and emotional benefits of yoga have been known for a long time, and regular yoga practice is recognised by the NHS in the UK as being an effective way to improve flexibility, balance, and strength. It can also be helpful in improving posture, and this has a positive effect on mood as well as physical health.

SELF-HELP TIPS

Yoga can be helpful in managing POP, when practised under the supervision of a suitably qualified and experienced teacher. The following postures are recommended:

the Shoulder Stand (*Salamba Sarvangasana*) or a modified version of it

the Pose of Eight Curves

the Boat posture (*Navasana*)

gentle breathing practise (*Mula Bandha*)

The following should be avoided:

full back-bend postures like the Wheel (*Chakrasana*) or the Bow (*Dhanurasana*)

vigorous breathing exercises (*Kapalabhati* or *Bhastrika*)

Chapter 4

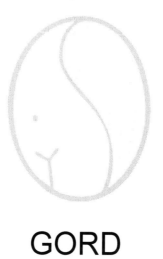

GORD

GORD

GORD is the short and snappy medical acronym for gastro-oesophageal reflux disease. This is a general term which covers a number of conditions, but they share one main symptom – acid reflux, where acid from the stomach rises up into the oesophagus (the gullet) and causes a painful burning sensation in the upper abdomen and chest. It is more commonly referred to as heartburn.

Why do I digress onto this topic here? I mentioned in the previous chapter that acid reflux was making it impossible for me to do a proper Shoulder Stand, even though this yoga posture would have been beneficial to my prolapse condition. In fact it was making movement of any kind difficult as it could be triggered so easily. Even walking about could make me feel queasy, and any position which affected my stomach directly – such as lying on my front, or bending forwards – could make me feel very sick indeed. At other times there was no obvious cause: I would wake in the middle of the night with a burning pain in my chest, and my stomach feeling knotted like a tight fist. If the rush of acid reached my throat it would set off a coughing fit which put considerable pressure on my weak and damaged pelvic floor. All this added significantly to the discomfort of the prolapse, and did little to improve my mood or sense of general wellbeing.

The curious thing was that all this started only three months before the prolapse occurred. Were the two connected? Mary thought they could be, the displacement of my womb and bladder throwing my digestive tract out of kilter. After all, neither my bladder nor my bowel was functioning at its best. The GP thought they probably were not connected, though when I asked her about it she did say, "Well, I suppose if you want to look at it holistically, they might be...." But her suggestion was that bacteria called H. Pylori* might actually be the cause.

Blood test results proved to be inconclusive, so I was referred for a gall bladder scan, and a consultation with a gastrologist to discuss having an endoscopy (a camera or "magic eye" inserted into my stomach), all to try and establish what was causing the excess acid. In the meantime I was prescribed *Lansoprazole*, a proton pump inhibitor which reduces the amount of acid produced. These capsules had the effect of reducing the symptoms noticeably as soon as I started to take them. Within a few days I was feeling a lot better, and looking better

* According to Patient UK (patient.co.uk) "Infection with H. pylori is the cause of most stomach and duodenal ulcers. H. pylori also causes some cases of non-ulcer dyspepsia".

too; my face lost its pallor and regained a healthier colour, while the whites of my eyes lost the yellow tinge they had acquired over recent months. I was surprised at the difference, as I had become accustomed to looking weary and jaded. Clearly we use the expression "off colour" for good reason! I certainly had been.

Most significantly, I could move better in yoga now that my stomach felt more comfortable, and could gain more benefit from the postures. This in turn made room for improvement both to the prolapse symptoms, and to the function of my digestive system. Getting treatment for the acid stomach was a huge relief, and made me feel that I was at last on an upward spiral.

When I went for the gall bladder scan a couple of months later the results were clear, with no sign of the suspected gall stones. By the time I got to see the gastrologist (nine months after I was referred and put on the waiting list) the symptoms were well under control and he signed me off, seeing no need to investigate any further.

It may well be pure coincidence, but as the pelvic organ prolapse condition improved, the heartburn subsided too. After taking the medication for six months I was advised to halve the dose, and did so successfully. Another six or seven months on, and I was able to take it every two or three days rather than every day, and soon I was only taking it every couple of weeks when the symptoms occasionally returned. The last batch of prescribed *Lansoprazole* has remained in my medicine cabinet, unused.

SELF-HELP TIP

Consult your Family Doctor about any health issues that might be hindering your recovery, or making it more difficult to manage POP

Chapter 5

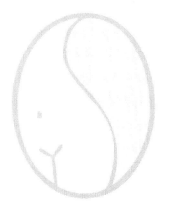

THE
EMOTIONAL SIDE

THE EMOTIONAL SIDE

I was learning a great deal about my body and how I could help it to cope and recover. But there was an emotional dimension to this which I needed to address as well. Putting on a brave face and swallowing my feelings was taking a lot of energy and concentration, and creating physical tension which was unhelpful.

To understand what I mean, try this little experiment:

o   Put on a frown.

o   That's it! Now frown some more.

o   Clench your jaw as well. Now lift up your arms. It's quite difficult to move them, isn't it?

o   Now relax your face, and smile.

o   Lift your arms again. You will probably find they move much more easily (and move further) this time.

How we feel affects the way we move, and vice versa – our physical state affects the way we feel.

I could tell that my loss of strength and my altered physical health were affecting my mood. In my vulnerable and weakened state I was unconsciously adopting a hunched and stooping   stance, whether sitting or standing, which friends and family noticed and commented on. I had looked like that in the past when I had been ill with depression. It is difficult to feel happy and confident in a permanently hunched position. Try it and see!

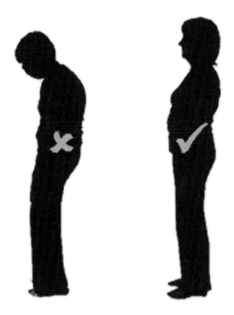

I knew I could be at risk of getting depressed again if I didn't handle this situation carefully. Having been through an episode of clinical depression ten years before, I was aware of the warning signs. So besides confronting the prolapse condition, I knew I had to confront the way I felt about it too. I loosened my grip, and allowed myself to cry. I encouraged myself to explore my feelings, and consider what was upsetting me so much about all this.

A lot of it was to do with facing up to my age, and with that, the awareness of my own mortality. I had managed to avoid that up to this point in my life. Now I found myself beginning to take on board the obvious but uncomfortable fact that I will not always be here. I could only creep around the edge of that huge issue, and take an occasional peak at it with all its implications.

More immediately worrying was the fact that I had lost all my physical confidence, and parts of my body were making it very clear that they were out of my control. I no longer knew for sure what I was or was not capable of; or what I could or should attempt to do if there was no-one with me to whom I could turn for advice. Previously I had always been physically fit, able to train up to do anything I wanted to do. I used to feel invincible. I didn't feel like that any longer. I was learning to accept a different version of myself, and having to face the fact that my body would fail me, in the end.

My womb and vagina were compromised, and this was having a profound effect on my self-image, my femininity, and even my sense of purpose and self-worth. I found myself experiencing feelings similar to those that I had been through when I had had a miscarriage, many years before; similar feelings of guilt, shame, and failure, and of wanting to hide myself away. Perhaps this was because physically I was responding in a similar way, feeling so vulnerable and self-protective. But perhaps it was because now, as then, I could find several reasons to blame myself for what had happened to me. And I do guilt rather well.

My internal dialogue went like this:

"I should have known something was the matter. I had twinges of pain and stiffness in my lower back for a few weeks before I discovered I had a prolapse. And I had been caught short a couple of times lately, barely making it to the loo in time. Wasn't that a clue that something was affecting my bladder? And why should my back be stiff, when I do so much yoga? I ought to have got all this checked out sooner!"

And it would continue, delving back into the past:

"I could have prevented this. It's all my own fault. I didn't look after my pelvic floor. I didn't even find out what or where it was, exactly. I was told to exercise it after I had had my babies, but I soon forgot about it. How could I have been so careless? And I've often been constipated but never worried about straining – I just assumed my body was built to cope

with such things. How could I have been so thoughtless? If only I had realised how important it was! All that long-distance walking I used to do, and the marathon-running – that won't have helped either. What was I trying to prove? I should have had more sense..."

And so on.

But there was really no point in beating myself up with "shoulds", "oughts", and "if-onlys", or bullying myself with hindsight. The fact is that with this condition, as with many others, the symptoms can creep up on you gradually, and become accepted as part of the way things are. The stiff back could easily have been a temporary muscular problem. As for the occasional leakage, a friend of mine who was a midwife back in the 1980's told me then that more sanitary towels were being bought to cope with incontinence than to deal with menstruation. Heaping blame on myself would be pointless and unreasonable. What mattered at this point would be how I responded to the situation as it now stood, and what steps I was to take going forward.

While I was being hard on myself, others around me were being kind. I was touched by this, but for some reason I found it difficult to receive it and accept offers of assistance. Being helped and allowing this to happen was all part of this new learning curve though. I would just have to alter my mind-set and adjust my automatic responses.

I recognised this when I arrived at the dental surgery one morning. The waiting-room was full. A white-haired gentleman stood up politely to give me his seat.

Normally I would have said quickly, "Oh, no thanks, I'm fine."

This time I knew I needed to accept his kind offer, and did so; just as earlier that day I had accepted a friend's offer to carry my shopping basket for me. On both occasions, accepting help made me feel lazy and rude. But isn't it perhaps more rude *not* to accept the helping hand, and to spurn the offer of kindness?

More than this – I was learning to ask for help when I needed it. When I was young I used to think that asking for help was an admission of weakness. Now I realise that it is actually an indication of strength to recognise when I need help and be prepared to ask for it. After all, I might cause more trouble for myself and others in the longer term by struggling to cope on my own. I have discovered that people usually do not mind being asked at all, and are only too happy to help when they have understood that they are needed. For instance, realising that my laptop was too heavy for me, I mustered up the good sense to ask a colleague if he would mind carrying it for me. I only needed to ask him once.

Accepting help might have been hard, but accepting sympathy was even harder; probably because it easily reduced me to tears, which was embarrassing. I learned to accept sympathy, though. I needed to receive support, and this helped me to be more kind and gentle towards myself. And I soon found that sharing my situation and feelings with others who cared had its unexpected benefits. Talking openly, especially with other women, helped me to get things in perspective and gave me hope. A lady in her seventies at one of the yoga classes, looking good and moving well, told me that she had had a failed operation for a prolapse condition thirty years before! And Mary had managed her own condition without having to resort to surgery.

If other women could come through this, strong and smiling, then so could I! I began to see the potential in the life-change I was having to go through, and became curious. Who would I become? What butterfly would be emerging from this particular chrysalis? She would surely be wiser and more experienced. And what more besides these new skills would she have to offer?

Curiously it has been observed in shamanic cultures that, traditionally, women undergoing some form of transformation or period of transition have strong feelings in the womb.

KEY INFORMATION

The emotional aspects of POP are significant and should not be underestimated

POP can undermine your confidence, your femininity, your self-image and your self-esteem

POP can trigger grief symptoms such as guilt, anger, tearfulness and a deep sense of loss

POP can trigger depression and/or stir up deep-seated emotional issues.

SELF-HELP TIPS

There is no need to struggle alone – talk about how you feel, and accept help and support from others

Seek professional help to process difficult emotional issues – ask your Doctor for referral to a counselling service.

Chapter 6

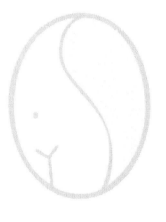

WAYS AND MEANS

WAYS AND MEANS

As I began to make sense of it all, I worked out some ways of doing things differently, to my advantage.

I realised that I needed to get plenty of sleep. This is, after all, essential repair time when the body can take a break from many of its activities and focus its recourses on recuperation. So rather than struggle against tiredness, I allowed myself more time for sleep.

I discovered that I was putting on weight, presumably as a result of being less active. I had called in at my local Weight Watchers meeting (having been a Gold member for several years) to buy their kitchen scales as a present for a friend. I had been hoping to drop in and come quickly out again with my purchase, unnoticed in the jostling January throng of new members keeping their New Year resolutions. But it was very quiet. I was recognised and welcomed, so I queued up to weigh. I was shocked to find myself so far over my Goal Weight that I now had to call myself a lapsed Gold member. So, as carrying excess body-weight is an issue with regard to pelvic organ prolapse, I made an effort to nip that potential problem in the bud. I made it a routine to attend my local meeting every week and to follow carefully their newly updated weight loss plan.

I adopted ways of tackling household tasks differently. I already had most of my shopping delivered, but I made sure I carried my goods from my doorstep in small quantities rather than in full, heavy bags. It took longer, but if my Tesco delivery man minded he never said so. I carried my washing to the line in armfuls instead of heavy basketfuls. I sat down to do the ironing or the washing up, or to chop vegetables. I progressed from being too scared to lift anything or stand for any length of time, to a place where I could sense whether or not I was putting undue pressure on my pelvic floor, and adjust my actions accordingly.

Sometimes doing things differently took nerve, as it meant being open about the problem. But I decided that it was worth being brave about this, as it has a positive side. The more people can be made aware of this issue, the more open we can all be about it. On one occasion, a friend looked askance at me when she had asked me to carry a large, full teapot from kitchen to table at a social event, and I said I could not do it.

"But it's not that heavy!" she exclaimed.

"It's not the weight," I explained, sensing an uphill struggle.

"It's the awkwardness of the action – having to lift the teapot away from my body because of its heat. I might hurt myself."

"Why not just try it and see?" she asked.

I had to explain that it was not as simple as that. I probably would not know that an unaccustomed action was going to do me harm, until the damage was done. There would not be a warning stab of pain – it did not operate like that. All I might notice would be a much more subtle feeling of discomfort; an awareness that things were not right. I had had to become very physically self-aware, listening carefully to my body and responding to its messages.

Luckily I had a strong network of supportive friends and family around me. One friend from a medical background asked whether I had been referred for gynaecological physiotherapy. I had no idea there was such a thing. Yes, she assured me, there are physiotherapists trained to work with clients on the specific muscles involved in supporting the pelvic organs. This made such good sense that I asked the next GP I saw to refer me. His response was that I would need to have the surgery first. I was disappointed, but I kept the idea in mind. It seemed such a sensible solution. Was there a hope that I could strengthen my pelvic floor to such an extent that I would not need surgery at all? I made a mental note to ask the consultant gynaecologist, when I eventually got to see one.

In the meantime, Mary suggested that wearing support pants might help. I tried them, fully supportive big pants from M & S. They were not as pretty as my usual little panties! But in my present circumstances, I found them so much more comfortable, and noticed a difference as soon as I started to wear them. I felt that I was no longer having to do all the work of holding everything in place, which actually gave me a chance to pay more attention to exercising and strengthening the pelvic floor muscles.

I began to carry myself better, and the improvement in posture had a knock-on effect on my mood.

My belly had become distorted by the changed position of my pelvic organs, so when I was wearing the support pants my shape looked better too. I began to get my confidence back.

A month after my initial diagnosis I went for a routine cervical smear test. I did not mention the prolapse, but the Practice Nurse soon found it. She asked if it was giving me problems when walking about, and suggested that wearing a thick pad would provide some support.

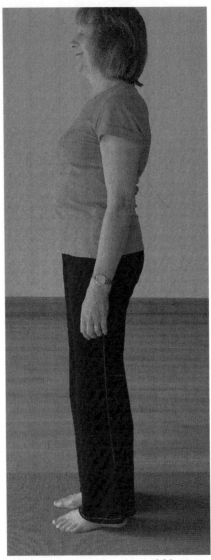

I began to carry myself better

This worked well, especially when held firmly in place by the support pants. I still had the feeling that a ball was descending through my vaginal opening, but at least I felt more certain that the ball was being contained!

Meanwhile, my bowel was creating problems of its own. It had become so sluggish that I was very constipated most of the time, which made me feel clogged and heavy. The GP had told me not to push to poo as this could make the prolapse worse. I tried prunes and bran for breakfast for a while, but they didn't make any difference. I tried using laxatives, but they felt like a harsh attack on my system. I talked to Mary about this one morning when she said I was looking pale in the YogaMobility class. She suggested I use *Fybogel*, which many of her students with health conditions use as it works more gently to ease everything through the intestine. I consulted my GP, who agreed that it could help. Within a day of starting to take *Fybogel* it seemed to be working, and my belly felt much more comfortable. I made some adjustments to my diet as well, drinking more water and making sure that I was eating plenty of fruit, vegetables and soluble fibre to help my intestine to function more easily.

I paid more attention to my bladder as well, cutting down on drinks containing caffeine such as coffee, hot chocolate, and tea. (Caffeine is a diuretic, which means that it makes you need to pee more.) And in circumstances where I used to just "hang on", now I would empty my bladder sooner rather than later to avoid putting it under unnecessary pressure.

Through conversations with friends and with professionals; through chance encounters; and through my own experience; I was gathering more and more pieces of practical advice and information which were making the prolapse easier to manage.

My belly had become distorted by the changed position of my pelvic organs, so when I was wearing the support pants my shape looked better too. I began to get my confidence back.

A month after my initial diagnosis I went for a routine cervical smear test. I did not mention the prolapse, but the Practice Nurse soon found it. She asked if it was giving me problems when walking about, and suggested that wearing a thick pad would provide some support. This worked well, especially when held firmly in place by the support pants. I still had the feeling that a ball was descending through my vaginal opening, but at least I felt more certain that the ball was being contained!

Meanwhile, my bowel was creating problems of its own. It had become so sluggish that I was very constipated most of the time, which made me feel clogged and heavy. The GP had told me not to push to poo as this could make the prolapse worse. I tried prunes and bran for breakfast for a while, but they didn't make any difference. I tried using laxatives, but they felt like a harsh attack on my system. I talked to Mary about this one morning when she said I was looking pale in the YogaMobility class. She suggested I use *Fybogel*, which many of her students with health conditions use as it works more gently to ease everything through the intestine. I consulted my GP, who agreed that it could help. Within a day of starting to take *Fybogel* it seemed to be working, and my belly felt much more comfortable. I made some adjustments to my diet as well, drinking more water and making sure that I was eating plenty of fruit, vegetables and soluble fibre to help my intestine to function more easily. Soluble fibre is found in oats, barley, nuts and seeds, and beans and pulses as well as in fruit and veg. It works more gently than insoluble fibre (wheat, wheat bran, corn, whole grains, and the tougher parts of fruit and vegetables such as the skins) as it makes stools softer and easier to pass.

I paid more attention to my bladder as well, cutting down on drinks containing caffeine such as coffee, hot chocolate, and tea. (Caffeine is a diuretic, which means that it makes you need to pee more.) And in circumstances where I used to just "hang on", now I would empty my bladder sooner rather than later to avoid putting it under unnecessary pressure.

Through conversations with friends and with professionals; through chance encounters; and through my own experience; I was gathering more and more pieces of practical advice and information which were making the prolapse easier to manage.

SELF-HELP TIPS

Get plenty of rest and sleep

Maintain a healthy weight

Avoid carrying heavy or awkward loads

Sit rather than stand

Control pants can help, perhaps with a pad for further support

Take care of your bowel. Avoid constipation by drinking plenty of water, and including plenty of fruit, vegetables and other sources of fibre in your diet. You might also need a gentle laxative – ask your GP for advice.

Take care of your bladder. Watch the amount of caffeine you drink, and don't leave your bladder too full for too long!

Chapter 7

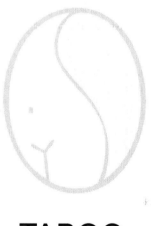

TABOO

TABOO

A male colleague was curious to know whether pelvic organ prolapse is a common problem among women, and asked me how many of the women I know have prolapse issues. I had to reply, "I haven't the faintest idea. Nobody talks about this."

Like miscarriage, it is a taboo subject. It was only when I miscarried myself in my early thirties that I took the time to find out how many women miscarry[*]. Until then, nobody had talked to me about it. It had been the same with depression. And now that I had a prolapsed womb and bladder, I realised that nobody had talked to me about that, either.

Admittedly, I could see why they had not. When I tried to talk about this situation myself, I realised how difficult that was. I struggled to find appropriate ways to explain my condition or to express my feelings about

---

[*] According to About.com, "Miscarriage in early pregnancy is common. Studies show that about 10% to 20% of women who know they are pregnant have a miscarriage some time before 20 weeks of pregnancy; 80% of these occur in the first 12 weeks. But the actual rate of miscarriage is even higher since many women have very early miscarriages without ever realizing that they are pregnant. One study that followed women's hormone levels every day to detect very early pregnancy found a total miscarriage rate of 31%."

it. Pelvic organ prolapse seemed too complicated, too personal; and very specifically female. A male friend whom I have known for a long time and know very well could see that I was struggling in the yoga class and asked me what was wrong. I felt I ought to meet his concern with an honest answer, but I found myself fumbling for words, and put it badly.

All I could find to say was, "My women's bits have slipped out of place."

He looked simultaneously sympathetic and baffled. I cannot explain exactly where the difficulty lay. Was I embarrassed to use words like *womb*, *bladder* or *vagina*? Or did I think he would be embarrassed to hear them?

There needs to be a change. Despite the awkwardness, the embarrassment, and the shyness, we must break the silence that still prevails over pelvic organ prolapse. How many women, I wonder, struggle with the symptoms of prolapse without asking for help? How many lack support from their nearest and dearest because they cannot bring themselves to mention the problem? And how many women delay seeking medical help because they are too embarrassed to talk about symptoms such as incontinence, even to their GP? Already physically unwell and emotionally vulnerable, these women risk feeling socially isolated too. We talk openly now about things like breast cancer, menstruation, menopause and pre-menstrual tension, which would have been taboo subjects in previous centuries of Western culture. We need to be open about pelvic organ prolapse and its related issues as well.

Let me remind you of the statistics: according to the BBC Health website, as many as half of all women who have given birth twice or more will have some form of pelvic organ prolapse. About one in every eight women over forty years old will have some degree of uterine prolapse. And the NHS reports that at least one third of adult women in the UK are affected by some form of the condition.

So we are all very likely to know – or to have known – many women with experience of pelvic organ prolapse, including those within our own families and social networks. I recently had a long conversation with a young friend (under thirty) who was experiencing problems in the pelvic area. We both found it equally difficult to talk about the subject, struggling to say words such as *uterus* and *vagina* in conversation. How odd that is! And how damaging such reticence could be! Would it not be so much more useful and healthy to feel free to share our experience, talk about these things openly and comfortably, and be better placed to give each other both practical advice and moral support?

Pondering on the embarrassment I had experienced and encountered, I got interested. I trawled through my contact lists, and put this question to all those women whom I dared to ask:

> *"What words do you use if or when you talk about your female parts – your womb, your vagina, and your bladder too – in a non-medical context? Do you feel able to say those words, or do you look for a euphemism to use instead?"*

I put this question to nearly forty women in my network of friends and family, whose ages ranged from twenty-four to seventy-three. They did not all respond, and I was not surprised – this just helped to demonstrate the point I was exploring. The replies I did get were fascinating.

"Women's bits" was the most commonly used expression, followed closely by "lady bits", "lady parts", "naughty bits" and even "wobbly bits". Some of my respondents came up with something more poetic ("tunnel of doom"); more descriptive ("womb and tubes"); or more euphemistic ("the under-carriage"). One invented words for these body parts when she needed to, coming up with terms like "floo-icky-walla" and "ooja-ma-flaj". One respondent in her twenties pointed me in the direction of the Urban Dictionary, where the definition given of the pubic area of a woman is "lady garden"; a phrase which to me sounded surprisingly coy.

Age did not seem to be a significant factor. These responses came from across the whole age range, and the younger women seemed just as uncomfortable as the older ones about using the words "womb", "vagina", or "bladder" in public.

What chance do we have of talking clearly and frankly about such intimate problems as pelvic organ prolapse if there is a taboo against using the most appropriate vocabulary? It is hardly surprising that many women still suffer in silence, with the result that the people closest to them underestimate the problem – that is, if they are aware of it at all.

I often find myself thinking about my mother, my grandmothers and the other women in my family who are all long gone, and wish I could talk to them about this very feminine problem. I feel a strong connection with them just now, and with other women in ages past and places distant who have had fewer recourses to draw on than I have. In ancient shamanic societies women worked through feminine issues together; menstruation, childbirth, miscarriage, menopause, prolapsed, and more besides. This is a skill and a strength that we seem to have lost in our modern, "civilised" Western culture. Can we recover this, I wonder, by being more open with each other now?

Chapter 8

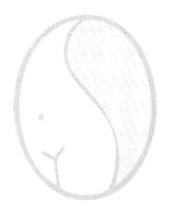

WHILE WAITING

WHILE WAITING

It took eight months to get an appointment with a consultant gynaecologist – more on that in the next chapter. But this was a blessing in a way, as it gave me time to work on managing the condition using yoga techniques, and to learn all the lessons and life-style changes that this experience had to teach me. I could have paid for a private consultation, but I chose not to. I preferred to wait, let time play its part, and see if I could mend this situation myself. It could be argued that I was being unnecessarily hard on myself. But for me, it worked out well. In fact, one of the things I learned was how to treat myself more gently than I had done when I was younger, and not to push myself so hard.

What else did I learn during this waiting period?

One big step forward in my personal development has been learning to accept the fact that I am aging – and that there are ways of responding positively to this. I cannot fight it of course, any more than Canute could hold back the waves. But I can accept it with acquiescence rather than resignation. Mirrors had begun to trouble me, with their unforgiving truths. My hair is greying, and I catch myself hunching sometimes, allowing my upper spine to curve and my shoulders to droop forwards. It is a sign of age, as well as a self-protective posture relating to the prolapse. But I am still able to stand with a perfectly straight back and raised breast-bone if I choose to. I do not have to concur or collude with this physical tendency; not yet. It will take a consistent and conscious effort not to, but this is an effort that I owe it to myself to make. Hunching can bring with it an array of physical and emotional problems.

Other signs of aging are less easy to tackle. But I am learning to accept what cannot be changed. One morning I noticed my aging hands in the sunlight falling on them from a window. The wrinkled skin no longer bothered me. I do not – and will not – look young any more. But I *can* look poised and elegant through having good posture and toned muscles. Regular yoga practice will determine that, and a balanced outlook to go with it. My later years do not have to constitute a period of decline. This can be a time of fruition – a time when all that I have learned and experienced during my life can be gathered together and developed to its full potential.

I find myself observing other women my age, and older, with new eyes. I am curious to see how they are responding to the issue of aging. Do they regard it as a challenge? Do they dread it like a curse? Do they fear it like a disaster? Or are they able to relish it as an opportunity for change, and a different outlook on life with different responsibilities and expectations?

Returning home from a foreign holiday in the spring, I was people-watching in the airport to while away the time. One woman fascinated me. She was sitting opposite me, with a beautiful but immobile face; smooth, pale skin; chestnut hair cut in a bob; and an upright posture. But her neck was like crepe paper, and her sandals revealed toes which were gnarled and starting to cross over each other. Her hands – and, incidentally, the man who sat with her – were similarly aged. Here was a woman fending off the effects of time, and perhaps resisting as well her transformation into the fruiting stage of life and the wisdoms it can bring. Looking at her, I recognised that I have some choice in this matter of aging. I can resist it: or I can welcome it.

"Why cling on so desperately to youth, to a self that exits in the past?" I mused. "Let it go! Just let it go! Allow these changes – and see what might come in its place!"

The other most important element in this new learning curve has been to experience a different level of empathy. I have discovered a little of what it is like to feel really old and to feel vulnerable. I have a better appreciation now of what it is like to have a disability, and to feel out of place among people who are (or who might appear to be) physically fit and healthy. One morning at YogaMobility I felt so weak and unwell that I had to be supported under each arm and lifted back up into a standing position at the end of the session. I hated having to be helped, and said so.

"Well, do you think anyone here actually *likes* it?" Mary asked.

I felt a surge of empathy with this group of physically challenged people, and was overwhelmed by it, humbled by their resilience, determination and humour. I had been working with them for some time, and had been under the impression that I understood how they felt. Now I realised how little I knew, and that I was only just beginning to understand. I was learning just a little of what it felt like to be disabled.

Mary said, "For you, this will mend. Your condition will improve, and you will recover. But you will never forget how this feels, will you?"

There is a saying that everything happens for a reason. If my suffering a prolapse had a purpose at all, it will have achieved much by teaching me this important lesson.

Chapter 9

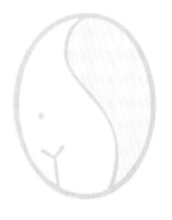

I MEET THE
CONSULTANT

I MEET THE CONSULTANT

A letter from the hospital arrived, offering me an appointment with a consultant in Gynaecology. As I sat in the waiting area I noted that it was eight months to the day since I had taken my first symptoms to the surgery on that snowy day just before Christmas. After eight months of waiting, I was to have ten minutes of consultation time.

The physical examination carried out by the gynaecologist produced some interesting results. According to the consultant, the GP had diagnosed a prolapse of the uterus and bladder. My bladder has prolapsed as well? I had not picked up on that. But remembering how shocked I was at the initial consultation with the GP she probably did tell me – I just had not taken in everything she said. However, the consultant was explaining that my uterus was no longer a cause for concern as the cervix was now much higher – almost back in its original position. All those techniques that I had learned and practised during the intervening months – they had worked! I no longer had a prolapsed uterus!

There was still a problem with my bladder though, as it was prolapsing through a tear in the pelvic floor. This was the bulge that I could still feel. I was given two options; surgery to repair the damaged muscle using a surgical mesh "patch", or a vaginal ring pessary (a soft plastic ring worn inside the vagina) to support the bladder. I did not like the sound of either of those options much. Surgery would be carried out under general anaesthetic, but success could not be guaranteed *. And there would be the risk of complications, such as infection, excess bleeding, or damage to the bladder or the bowel. To me the very idea of a surgical procedure in this area seemed like a personal invasion; and what impact would it have on my general health and wellbeing? Having a ring pessary inserted would be a less invasive procedure, but the pessary would have to be changed at the hospital every three or four months, and that would have to be done routinely for the rest of my life. The risks associated with ring pessaries included urinary tract infection, and ulcers.

I remembered the suggestion of gynaecological physiotherapy. I had noticed on the way in that the

---

* According to an article on the NewsMedical.net website, "Research conducted by the Pelvic Floor Disorders Network, an initiative funded by the National Institutes of Health, has revealed that the long-term success rates of surgery to treat pelvic organ prolapse are lower than expected. Nearly one-third of women develop anatomic or symptomatic treatment failure within five years of undergoing sacrocolpopexy for pelvic organ prolapse, according to a study published in the May 15 2013 issue of JAMA".

Physiotherapy Department in the hospital was on the same floor as Gynaecology, just along the corridor in fact. I pointed this out, somewhat desperately, as part of my argument in its favour! Could I possibly try this option instead?

The consultant agreed to refer me for physiotherapy to "give it a try – but give me a ring if you change your mind," she said.

I came away with another appointment made for the following February, when I would be asked again which option I wanted to take – the ring pessary, or the surgical repair. So which would it be? The devil, or the deep blue sea?

"Why don't you just have the operation?" a friend asked me later, conversationally, as she handed me a cup of tea. Just? *JUST!?*

So once again I was waiting, this time to see the physiotherapist. I explored various information websites to find out more about the treatment options and their potential side effects. I was not reassured. Still, by this time I had become curious to know how women in the past had handled pelvic organ prolapse, as surely this was nothing new. So I turned my attention in this direction to while away the time.

Apparently, the first written reference to uterine prolapse which has been found so far is in an Egyptian papyrus dating from around 2000 BC! The use of pessaries may go back as far as this, though the first description of a pessary appears in the writings of Hippocrates, a famous physician of Ancient Greece, who was alive around 460 – 370 BC.

The word "pessary" comes from the Greek "pessos" (or Latin "pessarium"), meaning an oval-shaped stone. (How comfortable does *that* sound??) Pessaries of various sorts have been used throughout human history to try to support the prolapsed uterus or bladder, ranging from a half pomegranate to oval shapes made from wool, linen, wood, cork or metal. The modern pessary evolved as new materials were discovered, but the principle has always remained the same.

Though clearly widely used, the pessary was not the only form of treatment recorded for pelvic organ prolapse. One less practical method of treatment that I read about involved approaching the prolapsed organ like a creature with a mind of its own, and making attempts to frighten it back into position! The Greek physician Euriphon of Cnidos (fifth century BC) recommended treating uterine prolapse with "succession", which involved hanging the woman by her feet from a wooden structure and shaking her up and down for a few minutes, then leaving her there for up to a day. Nice!

The physician Soranus of Ephesus was Greek but worked in Rome during the first part of the second century AD, and wrote a book entitled "Diseases of Women". In one account, he described removing a prolapsed uterus that had turned black. His recommended treatment for uterine prolapse was to bathe the exposed part of the uterus in warm olive oil, then gently push it back into place with a tampon made from wool wrapped in clean linen and soaked in diluted vinegar. The tampon then remained in the vagina to support the uterus, and the woman's legs were tied together to keep everything in place during the three-day healing process, after which time the tampon was removed.

Over the centuries, it seems, little changed. Surgery remained quite primitive and was rarely attempted for pelvic organ prolapse. Surgical repairs became more widely practiced from the early 1900's onwards, based on principles used in the previous century for treating hernias; but vaginal repair was not routinely carried out until the 1990's.

Having read all this, I felt very fortunate to be living in the 21st century.

KEY INFORMATION

Treatment options:

Surgical repair using a mesh "patch"

Insertion of a vaginal ring pessary

Gynaecological physiotherapy

Chapter 10

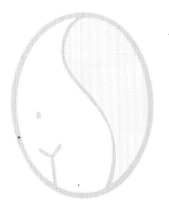

I MEET THE PHYSIOTHERAPIST

I MEET THE PHYSIOTHERAPIST

Less than three weeks after the consultation with the gynaecologist I was back at the hospital, in a group session with the physiotherapist. This was an information session on pelvic organ prolapse, in preparation for the gynaecological physiotherapy treatment. I looked around the room as I waited for the session to start. I was surprised to find that I seemed to be the oldest woman there. A young woman sitting near me had her baby on her lap. Another young woman in the row behind me was talking about how her prolapse had interfered with her training schedule for marathon running. While age can be a factor in prolapse conditions, it is clearly not the only one. Any woman of any age, it seems, can experience uterine or bladder prolapse.

The physiotherapist was welcoming and her pleasant manner put me at ease. She explained to us all in graphic detail, using a scale model, the workings of the pelvic floor and the relative positions of the pelvic organs in prolapse. I wished I had known all this before. I had had no idea that the pelvic floor muscle – or group of muscles – was so big, or so important, or that it had so much work to do. I found myself thinking that if I had known, I would most certainly have taken better care of mine. She described the basics of pelvic floor exercise, which involves contracting and relaxing the pelvic floor muscles to strengthen them. These muscle movements are sometimes called Kegel exercises, after the American gynaecologist Dr. Arnold Kegel who first devised them in 1948.

I braced myself to ask a question which was really important to me, and hoped against hope for a positive reply.

"Is it possible to avoid surgery by working hard to strengthen my pelvic floor?"

"Yes," she said.

Yes.

"And you need a strong pelvic floor even if you do have surgery. Repairing a tear in weak muscle is like mending an old piece of cloth – the next time it is put under any strain it will just tear somewhere else. Surgery should be the last resort".

At last I was hearing the answer I had been looking for; that I could potentially sort out this problem myself at source, by working on my pelvic floor.

"Why aren't more women with pelvic organ prolapse referred for physiotherapy as a first option," I asked, "rather than being routinely sent down the surgical route?"

She gave an exasperated sigh. "I wish I knew," she said.

She gave some advice about self-care to alleviate our symptoms, pointing out that there were other factors we could work on to enhance the effect of the pelvic floor work. Most of this I had already learned and put into practice through yoga, but there was an interesting point about toilet use. In our "civilised" Western culture, we have forgotten as adults how to sit on the toilet seat in a way which evacuates the bowel efficiently. A child on the potty has the right position instinctively; sitting with a straight back, feet apart, and leaning slightly forward, bending at the hips to ease out the stool without straining. And it is a natural process that takes time; it should not be rushed. I took this on board. How often had I rushed this in order to get it over with to get on with something else! I made a mental note to slow down, and to keep a book in the loo to help pass the time!

The physiotherapist proceeded to explain in more detail the exercises we would need to do in order to learn how to use the pelvic floor muscles and strengthen them, though she warned us that the effects would not be evident immediately – it might be three to four months before we saw any change. That did not surprise me. After all this was no quick-fix, but a long-term solution.

"How will I be able to tell whether I am contracting the right muscles?" someone asked. "How can I tell whether my pelvic floor is working? I can't see it – so how do I find it?"

The physiotherapist explained that the pelvic floor muscles are the ones we all use if we are trying stop ourselves from leaking urine, or passing wind. "Let's try that now," she suggested. Silence fell as we all concentrated hard, focusing on holding in an imaginary wee. Most of us were trying too hard: in the effort to tighten this one group of muscles there was a temptation to tighten everything. Several of us screwed up our faces, held our eyes tight shut, and held our breath too. "Don't forget to breathe!" she called. We laughed, and released our tension.

"Now let's try that again. Breathe normally throughout, and try to relax everything else apart from your pelvic floor. Make sure you are pulling up with the pelvic floor muscles, and not pushing down. Your tummy, bottom and thighs should be relaxed too." I realised that I had been clenching my buttocks – but that was not going to do the job. I had to concentrate on the muscles between my legs, at the base of my torso. That was better.

"Can you feel the muscle lifting upwards and forwards at the front? And at the back – around the back passage – can you feel it pulling inwards and upwards? If you are still not sure whether you are doing it right, you could try stopping the flow of urine while you are actually on the loo – but don't do this often, as it's not good for your bladder."

I could feel some pressure against my bladder and asked whether I should do the exercise lying down when I was at home. She advised that I should at first, and showed me (using the model and a small ball) how lying down would reposition the bladder during the exercise.

Once we had found our pelvic floors we practised tightening and releasing them, drawing up the muscles and then gently letting them go. We practised this a few times together. Once we had got the hang of this we were encouraged to try varying the speed, tightening a few times in quick succession, then resting the muscles; or tightening slowly before holding for a few seconds then releasing slowly, and resting again.

Now we were ready to go away and practise these exercises by ourselves, in preparation for our one-to-one physiotherapy sessions.

We were to work the muscles in two ways; slow holds to build up endurance, and short fast contractions to build power and strength. The fast contraction power exercise involved tightening the pelvic floor muscles, pulling up as hard as we could, and releasing them quickly. The idea was to build up to repeating this up to ten times in a row. This would improve the muscles' ability to react quickly when the pelvic floor is put under pressure by an unexpected cough, sneeze, laughter or a sudden burst of exercise.

The slow-hold endurance exercise involved tightening the pelvic floor muscles and holding the contraction for up to ten seconds, then letting go and relaxing the muscles for four seconds. The plan here was to build up to repeating this sequence (hold for ten, relax for four) ten times in a row. This would improve the overall strength of the pelvic floor and its ability to provide support to the pelvic organs.

I went home, and did my homework. I practised the exercises with an almost religious fervour and dedication. At first I counted the seconds as they ticked by on my watch; but as I progressed I found it more effective to notice how long a second lasted and learned to count the seconds ("one – and – two – and – three – and…..") at the right speed as they passed.

Following the introductory group session, I attended a series of one-to-one appointments with the same physiotherapist. I was shocked at my first session with her to find that I had no feeling in some areas of my pelvic floor. I used to think that I knew my own body well. I was so sure about this. And yet it just was not so!

I performed the exercises I had been practising, with the physiotherapist feeling my pelvic floor muscles from the inside. It was reassuring to find that I had been doing the exercises correctly, as I had to admit that it was difficult to judge this for myself. The muscles cannot be seen and can be difficult to feel if you are not used to being aware of them and exercising them, so having professional help is a huge advantage. But yes, I had been doing the pelvic floor exercises right and I had been doing them well, so I was making progress already. I was advised to move on from doing the exercises lying down to doing them standing, thereby working against gravity to make the pelvic floor work harder and strengthen the muscles more.

I continued to practise, increasing the number of repetitions and building up to going through the slow-hold sequence four times a day, and the fast contraction exercise at least twice a day.

To help me to focus on the exercise while I was going through the slow-hold sequence, I devised this "finger-hold" technique:

o   During the first slow contraction, I would grip the little finger of my left hand with the thumb and forefinger of my right while I counted the seconds of the contraction.

o   During the four seconds of rest, I would let go and move on to my ring finger, gripping this during the second contraction while counting...and so on.

This routine helped me to concentrate on counting the seconds spent holding the muscle tight, while keeping track of the number of repetitions at the same time. I would go through this sequence at quiet times, while watching television for instance, or while in the passenger seat of a car. Although it seemed to take a long time to go through, in actual fact holding the muscle tight (and my finger at the same time) for ten seconds, resting for four seconds, and repeating this ten times (i.e. using each finger one at a time) took less than three minutes to complete. And there was, of course, no need to feel self-conscious about doing these exercises, as no-one could see that I was doing them!

I could even use the "finger-hold" concentration technique described above without attracting any attention.

To make sure I practised every day I kept track of my pelvic floor exercise routines on a chart.

To make sure I practised every day I kept track of my pelvic floor exercise routines on a chart. At first I recorded the time of day when I did the exercise: later I found it more useful to record the number of repetitions. As the muscles grew stronger, and as I became more aware of them, I was able to get into the habit of contracting them whenever I was about to cough, lift something, or do anything else which would put any pressure on my pelvic floor. I could feel that pulling up the muscles both before and during the activity was helping to strengthen them and protect them from further damage.

I saw my physiotherapist once a month over the next few months. At each appointment she was very pleased with my progress. But then, I had worked hard. At the sixth appointment, after four and a half months of supervised pelvic floor exercise, she discharged me. My pelvic floor was strong enough to do what it had to do, and her work was done.

Just over a year had passed since I had been diagnosed with pelvic organ prolapse.

SELF-HELP TIP

To avoid straining on the toilet, sit with a straight back, feet apart, and leaning slightly forward, bending at the hips to ease out the stool. And remember that this is a natural process that takes time – so be prepared to allow time for it.

PELVIC FLOOR EXERCISES

N. B. Before you begin these exercises, consult with your GP or physiotherapist to check whether these exercises are suitable for you.

Getting started

To find your pelvic floor muscles, imagine that you are trying to stop yourself from having a wee. You should feel the muscles lifting upwards and forwards. If you find this difficult, try actually stopping the flow of urine when you are on the toilet (but don't do this often – holding back urine can put undue pressure on the bladder).

Now imagine you are preventing yourself from passing wind. Be aware of the muscles pulling inwards and upwards around the back passage.

Make sure it really **is** the pelvic floor that you are contracting, and not the muscles in your tummy, bottom or thighs. And make sure you are **pulling up** with the muscles, **not pushing down**.

When you have found the pelvic floor, practise tightening it and releasing it – drawing the muscles upwards and inwards and then gently letting them go. Repeat this a few times.

As you become more accustomed to the exercise try varying the speed. Tighten a few times in quick succession, then rest. Or tighten slowly – hold for a few seconds – then release slowly. Rest for a few seconds. Repeat.

Fast contractions exercise

Tighten the pelvic floor muscles, pulling up as hard as you can. Release quickly. Build up to repeating this exercise up to ten times in a row.

Slow contractions exercise

Tighten the pelvic floor muscles and hold the contraction for up to ten seconds. Let go and relax the muscles for four seconds. Build up to repeating this sequence (hold for ten, relax for four) ten times in a row.

You might prefer to try these exercises lying down at first to help you to focus on the muscles. As you become more used to it and as the muscles get stronger and more supportive, you will probably be able to do the exercises sitting, standing, or while you are active. **If you are in any doubt, consult your GP or physiotherapist.**

Don't hold your breath as you tighten the muscle – just breathe normally.

Make it a routine to perform these exercises at least twice a day.

Stay with it! These exercises are no quick fix – it may be three to four months before you notice any results.

The Finger-hold Technique
To help focus on the exercise during the slow-hold sequence and keep track of your repetitions:

Tighten the pelvic floor and hold the contraction

Grip the little finger of your left hand with the thumb and forefinger of your right

Count the seconds of the contraction ("One and two and three and...") up to a maximum of ten

Relax the muscle and let go of your finger

Count four seconds while you rest the pelvic floor muscles

Move on to your ring finger – grip it with your right hand, contract the pelvic floor, and count as before

Relax the muscles, let go of your finger, and count four seconds

Move on to your middle finger....and so on

Work towards going through this sequence ten times altogether, as you squeeze each finger and thumb in turn.

Pelvic Floor Exercise Chart

Use this chart to remind you to exercise your pelvic floor several times a day, **ideally under guidance from your doctor or physiotherapist.**

Mark each box with a tick, the time of day, or the number of repetitions and how many seconds you held for – whichever is most useful for you.

"Fast" means tightening the pelvic floor briefly and letting it go, up to 10 times in quick succession.

Marking on this chart each exercise as you complete it will give you a great sense of achievement, as well as a strong pelvic floor!

The chart is available to download from the website at www.womensbits.org with a sample completed chart. Alternatively, you could draw up your own chart based on the example on the following page:

DAY/REPETITIONS	1	2	3	4	FAST 1	FAST 2
MONDAY						
TUESDAY						
WEDNESDAY						
THURSDAY						
FRIDAY						
SATURDAY						
SUNDAY						

DAY/REPETITIONS	1	2	3	4	FAST 1	FAST 2
MONDAY						
TUESDAY						
WEDNESDAY						
THURSDAY						
FRIDAY						
SATURDAY						
SUNDAY						

Sample pelvic floor exercise charts can be
found on the womensbits.org website

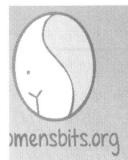

Pelvic floor e

Use the Blank copy o

Mark each box with a tick, the time of day, or the n

"Fast" means tightening the pelvic floor briefly and

Marking each exercise as you complete it on a char

** You should seek advi

Day	1	2
Monday	8.45	20.30
Tuesday	9.30	16.30
Wednesday	12.00	17.30
Thursday	8.30	11.45
Friday	7.30	10.00
Saturday	9.30	18.15
Sunday	9.00	13.45

Day	1	2
Monday	5 x 5	5 x 6
Tuesday	5 x 5	5 x 5
Wednesday	5 x 5	5 x 5
Thursday	5 x 5	5 x 5
Friday	5 x 5	5 x 5

Chapter 11

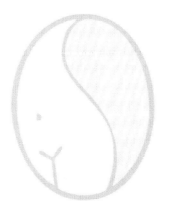

I SEE THE
CONSULTANT AGAIN

I SEE THE CONSULTANT AGAIN

My own work, of course, was not done. That would never be finished, if I wanted to maintain pelvic floor fitness – it had to be a life-long commitment. I continued with my exercise regime every day, and continued to record the exercises on my charts. I knew it would be so easy to let this lapse if I did not keep to a routine. Knowing that the alternatives were surgery or a ring pessary kept me focused and determined.

I kept doing my modified yoga, and put my feet up in the air when I needed to, though that need had become less frequent over time. By now I was feeling much better all round, both physically and emotionally. I had gone back to the YogaMobility classes after the Christmas break, this time as a helper again rather than as a participant. I also felt inspired to get to work on setting up my own website aimed at informing women about pelvic organ prolapse, and how it was possible to prevent, manage, and overcome it. I could feel some of my former energy coming back, and a desire to be more active and creative again.

I paid a lot of attention to my posture, and worked with Mary to improve it. I had learned to use my abdominal muscles. This was another area of my body that I thought I knew about, but did not. I had strong abs – I would not have been able to do the hill-walking that I had always done (and still can do) if I did not have strong abdominal muscles for support. But I had not been aware of them, and much of the time I had not been using them when other people would. For instance, I had not realised that they could influence the way I carried myself. I had been trying to correct my rather slouching posture for as long as I could remember, using my upper back and shoulders. How often did I hear these words when I was growing up?

"Stand up straight and tall! Shoulders back!"

But I had now discovered that if I used my abs and core muscles to stabilise the base of my spine, the rest of the spine would align itself effortlessly. No wonder my back had been so inclined to droop and hunch. It had simply been exhausted. Now that I could call my core muscles into play, the pressure - and the tension too - was off my back. Now I could perform movements in yoga (like lifting my arms and shoulders off the floor, from a prone position) which I had always assumed I just was not built to do. And I could stand up straight without so much conscious effort.

In the yoga classes Mary was working me hard, focusing on the upper abdominal muscles that I had been ignoring for so long. My posture was changing, as the muscles round my midriff were now starting to work to support my spine. My back was straightening, and my breast-bone was lifting. Exactly the opposite to what would normally be happening at my age! The ligaments in my upper chest had been starting to tighten and pull inwards, colluding with my habitual slouch to make it a permanent fixture. Now my chest was lifting into a more open position, and those ligaments hurt in rebellion as they were being repeatedly told to behave themselves!

You may be wondering why I have digressed to talk about posture. What has this to do with the pelvic floor? It has a great deal to do with it. The pelvic floor muscles – along with just about everything else - work a lot better if the head, neck and spine are in line with each other. Both common sense and personal experience tell me that.

I have already indicated that posture and mood are connected. I was also aware that a hunched posture has a negative impact on the digestive system and the breathing mechanism. What I did not realise until now was that restricted breathing affects pelvic floor function. The diaphragm and the pelvic floor work together, in synchrony. If breathing is shallow, the diaphragm cannot be fully functioning – and neither can the pelvic floor. So developing and maintaining good posture is not only relevant, but essential.

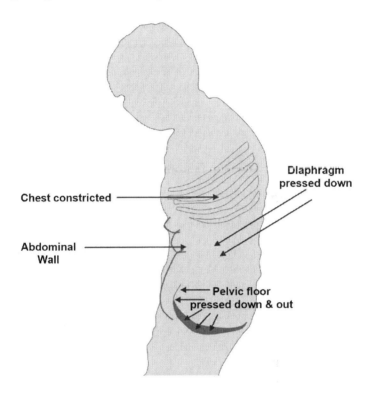

Chest constricted

Diaphragm pressed down

Abdominal Wall

Pelvic floor pressed down & out

Fourteen months after I was first diagnosed by the GP, I went for my second consultation with the gynaecologist. I was able to demonstrate to her that I was managing the condition using yoga, physiotherapy, and pelvic floor exercise. My upright stance was part of that demonstration.

"Your posture is very good," she said. "In fact, looking at you is making me sit up straight as well!"

I was able to report that I was now hill-walking, swimming, cycling, ice-skating, and doing yoga as before with hardly any need to modify my postures. I explained that I did not run or jump, I took care to avoid falling, and I avoided lifting heavy weights. But apart from those precautions, I was as good as new. She was so impressed that she discharged me on the spot.

"Just carry on with what you are doing," she said.

No surgical intervention then; no ring pessaries; no appointments or waiting lists. My relief was palpable. I had been discharged! Things could change, and I might need surgery at a later date if I were to have an accident, for instance, or if my muscles and tissues were to become weaker with age. I accepted that.

But for now, I was in charge of myself again.

SELF-HELP TIPS

Stay committed to doing your pelvic floor exercises regularly (at least three times a week) to keep your pelvic floor strong

Good posture helps both mind and body to function better, including the pelvic floor. It can make you look and feel younger too! Practising Yoga or Pilates - ideally with a suitably qualified and experienced teacher - can strengthen the core muscle groups which affect posture.

Low-impact exercise like hill-walking, swimming, and cycling can be very beneficial when managing POP

But avoid running, jumping, falling, or lifting heavy weights.

Chapter 12

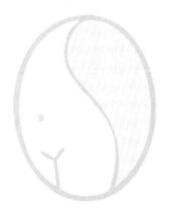

CATCHING THE RECOVERY MARKERS: A RECAP

CATCHING THE RECOVERY MARKERS: A RECAP

In the last chapter I mentioned hill-walking, swimming, cycling, and ice-skating. So far I have only talked about yoga. But as you can now see, I have been able to pursue other forms of exercise (with due care) despite the prolapse, and these have had a positive effect on my physical and emotional health and wellbeing.

So how had I fared on that fourteen-month journey from diagnosis to discharge from medical intervention? Looking back over that time, I can see that my recovery was not a steady progression. It was rather a two-steps-forward-one-step-back process, like an old dog climbing a steep flight of stairs.

Two months after the prolapse event and the diagnosis, I was starting to feel less unwell, more mobile and more positive. Even though my lower back was still feeling stiff and tight, I was generally feeling a bit more comfortable. The dragging sensation in my lower abdomen was less troublesome, and the feeling that everything inside was sagging downwards was less pronounced. I had been following all the advice described in the early chapters, and this seemed to be paying off. But my symptoms quickly returned if I got carried away and forgot to treat myself carefully. At times I just felt all out of kilter, as if my mind was still struggling to come to terms with my physical state and my emotions were scampering along behind trying to catch up. I would swing between feeling stronger and more positive, and feeling stiff and scared.

I have to admit that Fate – or Luck? - had a part to play. My husband, Nick, and I had a holiday booked to tour the archaeological sites of Egypt in March 2011, and had been looking forward to this for some time. I was concerned that this might be too gruelling for me now, involving too much travelling; too much time standing listening to tour guides; too much luggage handling and too little time to rest with my feet in the air. But not wanting to miss out on all those exciting, scenic and iconic places (not to mention the burst of mood-enhancing winter sun), I was determined to go.

However, on January 25th there were pro-democracy demonstrations in Cairo. By January 27th Tahrir Square was filled with people protesting against the thirty-year dictatorship of President Mubarak, and the mood was spreading to Alexandria, Aswan, Luxor and Suez. Egypt was poised for revolution. By January 29th, the Foreign Office was advising against any non-essential travel to Egypt, and encouraging British Nationals to leave. Our tour operator phoned to tell us the tour was cancelled, and to offer us a holiday elsewhere. The decision was being made for me. The Pyramids, the Nile, the Valley of the Kings.... they would have to wait until another time. My disappointment was tempered with relief.

We ended up going to Tenerife to explore its wild flowers and gardens from a base in Puerto de la Cruz. No touring; just colourful, peaceful surroundings and some warm sunshine. Much less taxing for me, and much more beneficial to my health and well-being!

The stay in Tenerife involved some gentle walking every day, as we explored the beautiful island with its rugged volcanic scenery. The exercise seemed to help strengthen my pelvic floor muscles. I was aware of being careful not to trip, but my anxiety diminished as my strength increased. By the end of the week, I felt more toned and my pelvic floor felt more supportive.

When we returned home I started going for walks in the country again – something I have always enjoyed doing, and which the GP had recommended as good, low-impact exercise for strengthening my pelvic floor without putting it under pressure. Walking at a steady, gentle pace made my muscles feel stronger, and lifted my mood as well. I had not realised how much the gastric reflux problem had been holding me back from being physically active. Going for these scenic walks was relaxing but energising at the same time, getting my system moving and demonstrating to me what my body was able to do, and thus increasing my physical confidence. With every day spent out walking my legs felt stronger, and so did my pelvic floor. I felt more at ease as I moved through landscapes steeped in history and mystery, taking in quiet hills, green headlands, and changing seas and skies. I absorbed as if through my very skin the distant views, the sights and scents of wild flowers and the sounds of lambs and bird-song. Walking in the countryside helped me to open out mentally and emotionally. I had not realised this before, but I could appreciate now that my prolapse condition had made me rather self-absorbed.

By this time three months had passed since the prolapse event and I was feeling more comfortable with it, though whether it was getting better or whether I was getting better at managing it I could not say for sure. My uterus seemed to keep shifting position – sometimes my movements felt constricted, sometimes not. But I knew by now that any discomfort was likely to be temporary. I just had to ease off a bit and wait for it to pass. There were many yoga postures and movements that I had been afraid to do for fear of causing damage. At this point Mary and I decided we should try things out rather than get stuck in a "can't do" attitude. Her advice to me shifted from "Don't do this movement" to "Do this if it feels all right to." She used this to teach me – and to remind the rest of the YogaMobility group at the same time – how easy it is to let disability become the status quo, rather than fight it. There is, of course, a fine line between fighting disability and pushing oneself too far, so it is vital to proceed with caution. Basically, if you believe that your body cannot do something, you will not even attempt it – and before long, your body will indeed be unable to do it. She got the whole class on their feet and moving that day – even some who find that very difficult – to prove her point. The physical and emotional habits that disability fosters can be very hard to break.

Another month went by. In addition to the regular yoga sessions and my country walking, I started swimming a couple of mornings each week. The GP had recommended this as good all-round aerobic exercise which does not put pressure on the pelvic floor. I had been putting this off as I am not very enthusiastic about swimming – especially that initial shock of cold water on the skin, that shiver that courses through the bloodstream!! But I enjoyed it once I was in the pool. The repetitive action was quite meditational and the time flew by. Like walking, going for a swim left me feeling both relaxed and energised.

By May I was quite clearly moving better in yoga. But where other activities were concerned, I still had to be patient. At a party with live music I was very disappointed that I was not able to join in the dancing. I just could not get my feet off the ground. I felt as if my pelvic floor would not be able to take the strain of any movement that had anything like a bounce in it.

There were still more lessons to learn about managing my condition, too. I knew from my first visit to the GP that I should not stand still for too long as this would put too much pressure on my pelvic floor; but I discovered that sitting for too long in the same position seemed to have a similar effect. And on a holiday in North Wales involving a lot of driving on rough country roads and tracks, I realised that I needed to make a conscious effort to pull up my pelvic floor while travelling in order to keep it safe.

By June I had to admit to myself that I was overdoing things, and was trying to rush ahead too fast. Much as I wanted to, I could not hurry the recovery process. I had to take things more gently and go back to spending more time resting with my feet in the air. Some of the discomfort I had felt in the early days of the prolapse had returned. Once again some of my yoga postures were restricted. I felt too delicate to go out walking. I could see that the muscles in my legs were losing tone. I felt frustrated and miserable.

Realising that I was on the edge of a downward spiral, I pulled myself up short just in time. I refused to be despondent, or to waste the progress I had made. I rested, but I went for short walks and an occasional swim too.

Gradually I regained my strength, but with an added awareness of the need to maintain all the habits which had assisted in my recovery so far. Imagine my joy when, at my son's wedding in July, I found that I was able to dance!

In September I started the physiotherapy programme which gave me a much stronger pelvic floor, and with that, a huge increase in confidence. Soon I had swapped the thick supportive pads I had been wearing for a thinner version. I found that I could manage without the backjack floor chair to support my back when doing seated postures in yoga, and could just sit on a wedge cushion to tilt my pelvis forward instead. This enabled me to sit comfortably with my head, neck and spine in line with each other – the ideal yoga sitting position for chanting and meditation. I did not need a thick cushion under my knees to be comfortable during yoga relaxation by this time either.

By December I was out on the hills doing what I call "a proper walk" of the sort I used to do when I was younger and fitter. It was a fifteen mile route in the Black Mountains and the weather was testing – high winds and freezing cold – so I was doubly pleased that I managed it without difficulty.

I was fired with renewed confidence in my fitness and strength. After several weeks of dismal weather I grabbed the opportunity on January 2nd to go ice-skating, and posted this message as my Facebook status:

> "*Enjoyed an exhilarating hour of ice-skating at Winter Wonderland this afternoon, in a rare spell of sunshine. I always love the Christmas skating, but missed it last year due to a health problem which I thought might rule out such activities permanently - so I'm a happy bunny today.*"

I was growing physically and emotionally stronger all the time, unfurling like a leaf in bud. By the following April - now sixteen months after my prolapse event - I was able to enjoy the thrill of a balloon flight. This was a sixtieth birthday present to Nick and to me, given the previous autumn, but at that time I was too wary to go. Now that I knew how to pull up my pelvic floor to brace it for a possible rough landing, I felt ready.

The evening of the flight could not have been more perfect. We climbed into the basket ready for take-off, and suddenly the ground below us was receding, the waving spectators getting smaller and smaller in the evening sunlight. We were gazing down on Raglan and its Castle, the Black Mountains, the River Severn and the Severn Bridges old and new, spanning the expanse of the tidal river. The experience was magical and surreal, like a dream. There was no sensation of movement, as we were drifting with the slight breeze – so no swinging or rocking, and no wind-chill either. All was warm sun, blue sky, and the ground four thousand feet below. No fear, no vertigo..... it felt as safe as houses. The landing on a rugby field brought us literally down to earth with a bump, the basket skimming a tree-top and tipping sideways as we came to a sudden halt! But all was well.

I remembered that during my first visit to the GP when all this started, she had suggested cycling as good aerobic exercise which does not put pressure on the pelvic floor, as this area is supported by the saddle. I got my bike out of the garage, where it had been left to rust since the prolapse. Cycling every week or two soon increased my fitness further, and had the additional benefit of strengthening my tummy muscles as well as my pelvic floor. By the end of May I had ditched the support pants apart from when I was exercising. Not only were my abdominal muscles stronger, but I think I had been getting lazy about using them and had been letting the big pants do all the work. There was an unexpected psychological effect too, in that I felt more like my old (or rather, younger) self in pretty underwear!

Of course I had to keep remembering to take care when handling weights, and I made sure I did not have to lift my bike myself. But by August I was pleased to find that I was now able to lift my rucksack onto my back to go for a day's walk, without having to ask for help. I carried out this action in two stages, by lifting the rucksack onto a chair, step, wall, or other intermediate surface first. I just had to remember to pull up my pelvic floor to strengthen it before carrying out the lifting action.

By this time I was able to move much more easily and gain much more benefit from my yoga practice. During the months following the first anniversary of the prolapse event, I had recovered enough flexibility and abdominal strength to do movements such as leg-raises; *Paschimottanasana* (a seated forward bend); and the Cobra (a back-bend posture). I could still feel some restriction when bending sideways - in the Triangle posture, for example. But I could now do full Shoulder Stand, on a good day.

In September I enjoyed an exhilarating walk in the Lake District of eight and a half miles with over 2,500 feet of ascent. We did a circuit from Haweswater, and covered several peaks including High Street, Rampsgill Head, High Raise, and Kidsty Pike. Names to conjure with. The weather was fine and warm, a remnant of summer lasting into the autumn days. The air was clear and the views were heart-stoppingly beautiful. I used trekking poles for stability, and came downhill slowly to avoid jarring. No problem. Nearly two years on from the prolapse, I had come back to myself again.

I stood on the hillside, arms outstretched, watching the swallows swooping and feeling as if I could fly too.

SELF-HELP TIPS

Be patient - recovery can be slow and not always steady

Be determined – but don't overstretch yourself

Be kind to yourself

Be aware of your pelvic floor and keep looking after it.

Chapter 13

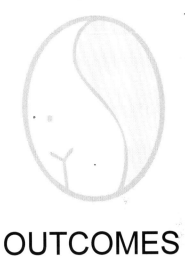

OUTCOMES

OUTCOMES

Recently I passed the third anniversary of my pelvic organ prolapse. I went ice-skating to celebrate. My activities are back to normal for me, with some modifications. No running, no jumping, and I do not lift anything that is likely to be too heavy for me to manage safely. I listen to my body, and think before I move. I am very aware of my pelvic floor and can tighten the muscles at will whenever a sudden movement – such as a cough or a sneeze – is likely to put them under pressure. My digestive system is functioning well now and I no longer take *Lansoprazole* or *Fybogel*.

I still do my pelvic floor exercises, every day. I do not follow a strict routine any more: I just do the exercises whenever I remember to. And rather than filling in charts, I started using the Tena Lady "my pff" app[*] on my phone. This took me through a sequence of "squeeze and hold" exercises; recorded how often I had done them; tells me how well I am doing; and reminded me to do them if I forgot. There is now a choice of pelvic floor exercise apps, several of them free to use. At the time of writing I am using Kegel Kat. This one gives

---

[*] http://www.lightsbytena.co.uk/my-pelvic-floor-fitness/app-info/

some basic information about pelvic floor (Kegel) exercises, takes you through some routines, and allows you to set yourself up to three daily reminders. It sounds or vibrates your mobile as a signal to squeeze or relax the muscles, so that you can go through the exercise sequence without having to keep your eyes on the screen. I find it quite fun to use.

During a recent visit to the GP surgery on another matter, I met the doctor I had seen when I was first diagnosed with pelvic organ prolapse. She told me that she now refers prolapse patients directly to gynaecological physiotherapy, and that this is gradually becoming more accepted as a general practice. This was very good news for me to hear indeed!

Mentally and emotionally, I am strong again. And I have been busy. In view of the difficulty I experienced when first diagnosed in finding useful information about POP – especially with regard to clear explanations, and the full range of treatment options and self-help available – I have compiled all the information I gathered from various sources, and put it together in one place where it can be accessible to other women wanting to find out more about how to prevent or manage pelvic organ prolapse. The result is the Women's Bits website www.womensbits.org which was launched in January 2013.

Women's Bits provides a wealth of information on the pelvic floor and how to look after it. It includes information not only to help manage a prolapse condition, but also to prevent it happening in the first place. Topics covered on the website range from symptoms and warning signs of the condition to campaign issues around its treatment; from pelvic organ prolapse in history to the treatment options currently available; and from how to exercise your pelvic floor to how to take care of your bladder and bowel. Womensbits.org will also be updated frequently with news and observations on pelvic organ prolapse-related issues.

Women's Bits is not a substitute for medical support, and neither is this book. But the fact remains that there is much that a woman can do for herself (especially while she is on the waiting lists for consultations and treatments) which can make the condition easier to live with, reduce its impact on her daily life and wellbeing, and even reduce or postpone the need for medical intervention or surgery. I am hoping that Women's Bits will also catch the attention of women who so far are not affected by pelvic organ prolapse, and will encourage them to be more aware of their pelvic floor and to look after it, perhaps thereby avoiding ever having to go through the physical and emotional effects of the condition.

Why have I called the website Women's Bits? Remember the chapter on Taboo, and the piece of research I carried out and recounted there? "Women's bits" was the most prevalent term, among the women I asked, that was used to refer to the female organs when a euphemism was called for – which, for far too many women, is all of the time.

If this book and the WomensBits.org website can help other women to manage and even overcome pelvic organ prolapse without going down the surgical route unless for them it is absolutely necessary, then I shall feel that my efforts will have been worthwhile. What is more - if my work can encourage women to be more open about female health issues, less passively tolerant of them and more mutually supportive about them, then I shall be leaving in my footprints the seeds of social change for our daughters, our grand-daughters, and beyond.

VISIT WOMENSBITS

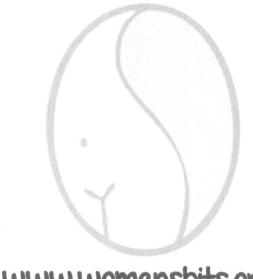

www.womensbits.org

VISIT WOMENSBITS

Women's Bits provides a wealth of information on the pelvic floor and how to look after it. It includes information not only to help manage a prolapse condition, but also to prevent it happening in the first place.

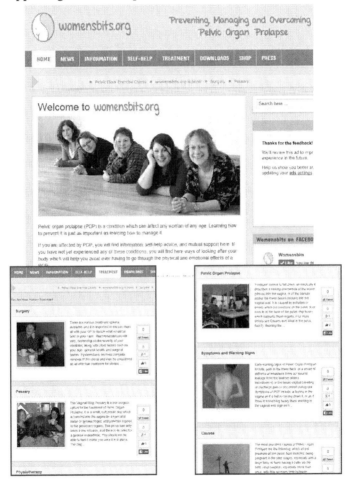

IF YOU FOUND THIS BOOK HELPFUL, PLEASE RECOMMEND IT TO OTHERS!!

Thank you for reading *Holding the Ball* I am sure you will find it useful both to you and to those who care about you.

If *Holding the Ball* was helpful to you, it will also be helpful to others. So please take the time to leave a review, so that you can help to bring this book to their attention and help them too.

RECOMMENDED READING

Books on POP:

Sherry J. Palm, 2009. *Pelvic Organ Prolapse: The silent epidemic*. Eloquent Books. New York.

Jenni Russell, 2012. *Pelvic Floor Secrets: 6 weeks to confidence, continence and sexual satisfaction*. Filament Publishing. Croydon.

Elizabeth E. Houser and Stephanie Riley Hahn, 2012. *A Woman's Guide to Pelvic Health*. Johns Hopkins University Press. Baltimore.

Christine Ann Kent, 2007. *Saving the Whole Woman: Natural alternatives to surgery for pelvic organ prolapse and urinary incontinence*. Bridgeworks.

Mary O'Dwyer, 2011. *Hold it Sister: The confident girl's guide to a leak-free life*. Redsok.

Books on Yoga:

Jaime Stover Schmitt, 2002. *Every Woman's Yoga: How to incorporate strength, flexibility and balance into your life*. Prima Publishing.

Linda Sparrowe and Patricia Walden, 2002. *The Woman's Book of Yoga and Health*. Shambhala Publications.

Kathryn Budig (editor), 2013. *The Women's Health Big Book of Yoga.* Rodale Books.

Lynne Robinson, 2010. *The Pilates Bible: The most comprehensive and accessible guide to pilates ever.* Kyle Cathie.

Books on emotional wellbeing:

Tim Watkins, 2013. *The Depression Workbook: 70 self-help techniques for recovering from depression.* Waye Forward (Publishing).

Tim Watkins, 2012. *Helping Hands: How to help someone else cope with mental health problems.* RPX Empire Books.

Tom Rath and Jim Harter, 2010. *Wellbeing: Five essential elements.* Deckle Edge.

Printed in Great Britain
by Amazon